Natural Remedies!

Natural Herbal Remedies And Beyond For Your Health And Natural Beauty!

I0419460

Sarah Brooks

STOP!!! Before you read any further....Would you like to know the secrets of Anti Aging?

If your answer is yes, then you are not alone. Thousands of people are looking for the secret to reducing wrinkles, looking younger, and maintaining a youthful appearance.

If you have been searching for these answers without much luck, you are in the right place!

Not only will you gain incredible insight in this book, but because I want to make sure to give you as much value as possible, right now for a limited time you can get full **100% FREE access to a VIP bonus Ebook** entitled **Anti Aging Made Easy!**

Just Go Here For Free Instant Access:

www.LuxyLifeNaturals.com

Legal Notice

Disclaimer Notice

the author and publisher reserve the right to alter and update the information contained herein on the new conditions whenever they see applicable.

Table Of Contents

Introduction

I want to thank you and congratulate you for purchasing the book, "Natural Remedies! - Natural Herbal Remedies And Beyond For Your Health And Natural Beauty!".

This book contains insight to the amazing world of natural herbal remedies and how incredible they can be for your health!

This day and age many people automatically turn to the traditional medical field for all of their health and beauty problems looking for the answers. Unfortunately, many times these solutions can also come with their own problems. Now you have two problems to be treated! The first one you were looking to take care and a myriad of other side effects you must now also treat.

Over the years I have began to realize that this is a very common and many people are looking for additional, more holistic ways of treating minor issues that won't have them second guessing later. This is my motivation for creating this book and hope you will find many solutions to everyday problems, and live a much healthier and happy life!

Thanks again for purchasing this book, I hope you enjoy it!

Chapter 1: Natural Herbal Remedies: An Introduction

I am so happy you have decided to go down this journey with me and I hope you find what you are looking for! I want to take a moment to explain why I have structured this book in the way it is. First this book is meant to provide you with as much information with as little clutter as possible, because at the end of the day what you want is solutions to your problems, not some fancy way of saying it! So please don't get hung up if you feel that sometimes the text is just giving you the facts and not a lot of fluff, that is the way it is designed - so you can get the most out of it! Now let's get started!!!

What's so great about using natural remedies, you ask? There are many great things about it, often overlooked by people who are quite used to taking medication that's been prescribed to them or ones that they are most familiar with. There's nothing wrong with that, of course, but one needs to be mindful of the different side-effects that these chemicals may bring about. Many people turn to the use of these natural remedies (otherwise known as home remedies or folk medicine) for many of their ailments because of the fact that these are made out of natural ingredients. Herbs, vegetables and fruits are just a few of the most common ingredients used in these remedies. The best bit, however, is that many of these things can be easily found in an average kitchen.

But will it work? Well, if you consider the fact that throughout history people have used and relied upon these natural medicines, then the answer would be a solid yes. This was before modern medicine was invented and the use of synthetic drugs was propagated. It works but as to what extent, well, that varies from one individual to the next. For simple cures, however, even some doctors recommend their use instead of depending on over the counter medicine. Even in the food that we consume on a daily basis, there are healing properties that can help combat certain types of illnesses. It would be to our benefit if we harnessed it and used to as supplements to the medications that we're taking. In fact, if it happens to be potent enough, you can use it by itself. Research and studies do prove that many of these natural remedies possess properties that work in the same manner as synthetic medication.

How do you get started with it then? Well, first off, you would require a certain knowledge of which ingredients you need for a particular ailment. That's where this book is going to come in handy. We'll get more into the specifics later.

Spices, herbs and even fresh food can be used effectively when it comes to treating most ailments that can range from minor pains to even infections. These days, people would rely on antibiotics for these things. Those can be quite expensive, let's be honest, and in some cases, they can also cause adverse side effects if misused. There's also the fact that these antibiotics also end up killing the good or beneficial flora and fauna in our bodies, thus making recovery time lengthier than usual. In worst case scenarios, they can backfire and actually damage our immune system. With natural home remedies, however, you can avoid all of that. Besides treating the infection itself, it also helps in strengthening our immune system which makes it more capable of defending itself from other ailments. We also recover better with it as it readily promotes mending and healing of various aches and pains, as well as burns and wounds.

Besides medicine, you can also make use of home remedies to make your own mouthwash and if you're really good, toothpaste. Some people go to the extent of creating medicinal soaps that allow them to avoid mass marketed ones that might contain ingredients that they're allergic to, don't support or extremely harsh for the skin.

It takes a bit more work to achieve these, but if you're really keen, a few hours out of your day should be enough. So, if you have certain skin issues and want to give natural soap a try, look to the later chapters for instructions on how you can make some. Besides hygiene products, you might also want to try creating remedies for indigestion and constipation, both common problems for modern man considering the diet we all have. This would be good if you need to regularly take something in order to be able to move your bowel easily.

What else can these home remedies be used for? There's also some that you can make in order to help yourself or a loved one recover from the flu in a quicker fashion. You may also make teas that would help relieve a cough or a sore throat. A throat spray (typically used for asthma) can also be made through the use of natural ingredients that, when compared to a store-bought one, would be far cheaper.

We've already touched on it but these remedies aren't just meant for internal use only. Besides the soaps and the mouthwash, you can also create your own natural cleanser that would treat skin conditions such as acne. An antiseptic spray made from natural ingredients can also be concocted and this would be great for eliminating dermatitis, as well as killing bacteria from scratches or cuts. It can also effectively heal blisters.

Needless to say, there is a lot that one can do when it comes to home remedies. All you really need is a simple guide, as well as a few free hours for research. The more familiar you are with the benefits of a particular ingredient, the better you will be at making and mixing remedies.

Chapter 2: Natural Brews For Coughs And Flus

When it comes to dealing with the common cough, there are many different natural remedies that have been proven effective for relieving its symptoms and speeding up the body's recovery. The best bit? Many of these ingredients can be easily found in your average kitchen. Shall we get started?

Thyme – Thyme, not many may know, is actually approved as a treatment for upper respiratory infections, coughs, bronchitis, as well as whooping cough in Germany. This comes with good reason, of course. Don't underestimate those little leaves for they are packed with countless compounds that are very potent when it comes to relieving cough. Basically, Thyme flavonoids help in relaxing ileal and tracheal muscles, both of which are involved when a person is coughing. Thyme is also known to help reduce any inflammations. Take it in tea form by mixing two teaspoons of crushed Thyme leaves to a cup of boiling water. Cover and let it steep for ten minutes, then strain before drinking.

Flax, Honey and Lemon – Okay, so this might not be the most delicious looking but don't disregard it just because of that. Boiling flaxseeds in water will result in a rather thick and gooey gel but this would be effective when it comes to soothing your throat, as well as your bronchial tract. Lemon and honey both act as mild antibiotics so when added to this syrup, it helps in making it super-soothing. So what do you need to do? Simply boil two to three tablespoons of flax-seeds in a cup of water until it becomes thick. After, simply strain it and add about three tablespoons of lemon juice and honey. Take a tablespoonful whenever you need it.

Brewed black pepper – Alright, this natural remedy is rooted in a couple of very different traditions: Chinese medicine and New England folk medicine. It can't get more different than that, right?

Well, the idea behind it is that black pepper actually stimulates the mucus flow, as well as circulation. By adding some honey to the mix, you're also adding a mild antibiotic which is also capable of reliving cough. To make the tea, you would need to place at least a teaspoon of freshly grounded black pepper and two tablespoons of honey in a cup. Fill this with boiling water and allow it to steep. Make sure you have it covered and leave it be for fifteen minutes. Strain after and sip on it whenever needed. This remedy would work best on wet coughs and isn't suitable for dry ones.

Lemon – Want something quick and easy? Well, this one isn't for the faint of heart, but it is very effective. All you need to do is quarter a fresh lemon, sprinkle generously with salt and black pepper, then suck on it. A simple and quick cough relief.

Now that we have coughs covered, what about the flu? After all, there is such a thing as "flu season" and one needs to be prepared for it. What natural remedies are available for this purpose?
Garlic – It contains natural anti-fungal, as well as antibacterial properties that can effectively kick any sickness out of your body. However, garlic does lose its potency when it's cooked so it would be best to eat it raw. Besides that, you can also try what's referred to as a garlic shot. Finely mince one to two cloves of garlic, put it in a small shot glass and simply down it in one go.

Coconut Oil – By now, almost everyone already knows of the many wonders of the coconut. Who would have taught that its oil has healing properties too? Well, because of the fact that it contains a naturally high level of lauric acid, which when converted by our bodies becomes a potent antimicrobial, it certainly is beneficial when it comes to boosting our immune systems and defending the body from illnesses. It can be eaten with food, taken straight out of the jar or melted into hot tea. Take your pick.

Fermented Cod Liver Oil – Because it contains high levels of Omega- 3, it becomes the ideal remedy for reducing inflammation, as well as boosting our immune health. It also contains vitamins A and D that are recommended during times of sickness.

Liquid Chlorophyll – Yes, I'm talking about the compound that makes leaves green. It is alkalizing which then makes it difficult for viruses to survive it. Besides that, drinking it can help purify our blood because of its high nutrient content. For daily consumption, simply add about a teaspoon of it to your water and drink it throughout the day.

Chapter 3: Headache And Fever Solutions

Nowadays, popping pills to get rid of a headache has become so common that nobody even questions the possible side effects that it might have. It's safe to say that yes, it does have certain side effects that happen with constant use. You don't always need to turn to synthetic medicine to get rid of your headaches, however. There are countless natural home remedies that you can make use of in order to alleviate the palpitating pain that comes with this nuisances. So, if you get a headache after work today, go on and try any of these:

Ginger tea – It has been used throughout Asia for centuries now in lieu of aspirins. All you need to do is crush up about an inch of ginger root and add it to boiling water. This should help reduce inflammation and takes about the same amount of time as an aspirin in order for it to take effect.

Capsaicin cream – This one can be made at home or simply bought from a natural remedy store. The active ingredient would be cayenne pepper and to use it, you would need to apply a small amount inside your nostril on the side of the head where the pain is in. What does it do? This cream blocks nerve pain signals, thus significantly lessening the pain.

Feverfew – In many clinical trials, it has been observed that this supplement from the sunflower family is quite potent when it comes to the treatment of the dreaded migraine. It helps in reducing inflammation, which then takes any pressure off of the nerves and can even prevent migraines entirely.

Mint Juice – Mint has antiseptic properties, as well as anti-pruritic properties that are beneficial when it comes to relieving headaches. Both menthone and menthol are great for this purpose, as well. To use it, you can use mint tea compresses on your forehead to alleviate any discomfort. You can also choose to apply mint juice on it, as well as on your temples to make it more effective. Along with mint juice, you can also try one that's made out of coriander.

Lavender Oil – The health benefits of lavender are quite well known. Did you know that it can also be used for treating headaches, as well? It's simple, all you need to do is add some lavender oil into a bow of hot water and inhale the vapors from it. Do this for a few minutes every day or whenever you need it. You can also opt to apply it externally to your forehead while massaging your temples. However, never ingest lavender oil orally.

Now that we have a few basic headache remedies discussed, what about the dreaded fever? For the most part and much like headaches, people would often take over the counter medication for it. It is effective, yes, but there are also safer natural home remedies that you can try whenever you're feeling under the weather. Here are a few suggestions:

Chamomile tea – This is one of the most popular varieties of tea and can do more than just induce a sense of calm and relaxation in people. It can also be used to help lower a person's fever. Besides that, it is also capable of treating cramps, muscle pain and anxiety.

Echinacea – Used for centuries by the Native Americans when it comes to the treatment of colds and flu. This herbal remedy can also help in boosting our immune system, thus making us less susceptible to sickness as well as eliminate the chances of your fever coming back.

Gingkgo – Otherwise known as ginkgo biloba, this popular herb is also a well-known remedy for fevers. Besides that, it is also known for its potency when it comes to improving brain activity, as well as body circulation. It is available in tea form, which makes it easier to ingest. Take it daily with your meals.

St. John's Wort – Often used as a natural alternative to prescription depression medicines, it also has the ability to reduce fevers and boost the immune system while it treats the body.

Chapter 4: All Natural Skin Remedies

The best thing about these natural herbal remedies is the fact that they can be used for a wide variety of purposes. From illnesses to certain skin issues, there's bound to be a recipe that should help you. If you've been experiencing certain skin allergies, bug bites and other things that have appeared and diminished the glow of your skin, then you'll certainly benefit from the following:

Bentonite Clay – Clay is great to use whenever you experience itchiness on your skin, as well as for treating acne break outs. It can also help when it comes to venomous bites and stings that you can get from spiders, wasps and bees. Basically, the clay draws out the venom from the skin, as well as alleviates the pain, thus allowing the area to recover quickly. How to use? Get some untreated clay which is also known as green clay. This would be the most potent kind and works wonders when it comes to healing the skin. Simply mix it with a cup of filtered water until the consistency begins to resemble peanut butter. After that, you just dab it onto the affected area. Wait until it dries and then peel it off.

You can also try doing a clay pack. For this, you would need to spread the clay on a clean piece of porous fabric. This could be cotton, muslin or even flannel. Afterwards, place the clay covered cloth onto the affected area. Make sure the clay is directly touching the skin. Keep it on for four hours or until the clay dries and hardens.

Apple Cider Vinegar – This might not be the first time you're hearing of the wonderful benefits that ACV has. It is a very potent antiseptic and also contains antibacterial and anti-fungal agents that would effectively relieve itching that's usually associated with dry skin. Take for example sunburns and dandruff. It is also popularly used for pets; all you need to do is add a cup of it into their bath water. You can also drop some of it onto a cotton ball, as well as a wash cloth then dab it onto the affected area. It would be best to use raw and unfiltered organic cider vinegar, the kind that still has strand like sediments floating on the bottom of the bottle. This is because you can rest assured that the bottle still contains all the raw enzymes that are beneficial for medicinal use.

Aloe Vera – Everybody knows this, aloe Vera is great for the skin. It is used for a variety of skin irritations, as well as for its ability to help sun burnt skin recover quickly. Besides being soothing to the skin, it can also relieve swelling and keeps it moisturized. It is a common compound used for natural lotions and creams. The best part? It is also a common plant. If you live in Southern California, then there's an 80% chance that there's one growing in your yard. How to use it? Simply break off a leaf and carefully cut it open in a lengthwise fashion, from top to bottom. Scoop out the gooey gel that's inside it and rub it directly onto the skin. If there's some left over, then refrigerate it. It should keep for a week.

Chapter 5: Natural Remedies For Anxiety And Stress

Under a lot of stress? Feeling anxious for no reason? Well, instead of taking prescription medicine which can damage your internal organs in the long run, why not try something more natural? This way, you're not just curing your anxiety or stress issues. You're also giving your body nutrients that would help boost your immune system further. You know what they say, a healthy mind and a healthy body make for a productive individual.

So, what are some of these herbal remedies?

Green Tea / L-theanine –Buddhist monks in Japan are capable of meditating for hours on end while remaining alert and relax. One of the reasons as to why they are able to do this is attributed to the tea they drink. Green tea contains an amino acid known as L-theanine which effectively curbs a person's rising blood pressure and heart rate. There have been studies that show how it was able to help calm down subjects that are prone to anxiety just by taking a 200-mg dose of it beforehand. Drink tea with every meal or with every snack and you should be able to consume enough of it for the L-theanine to take effect.

Hops – The beer you drink contains it as well but when brewed, you wouldn't get the same tranquilizing effects of this bitter herb. It has a sedative compound which is a very volatile oil and as such, it is only available in tinctures and extracts. If you look around, then you'll easily find aromatherapy products with it as a base. It is bitter so mix it with some chamomile or a bit of mint if you're planning on drinking it for tea. It would help promote a peaceful night's rest.

Valerian – There are certain herbal supplements that are very effective when it comes to minimizing anxiety, but without needing to make you sleepy whilst there are those that are meant to sedate. Valerian offers help to people with sleep problems including insomnia. It does contain a sedative compound so it falls under the latter category. The plant's smell isn't the most appealing and for this reason, people prefer taking it in capsule form or as a tincture instead of taking it as a tea. Remember, it will make you feel sleepy so take it at night. Make sure to avoid taking it prior to heading to your work as it induces sleepiness.

Lemon Balm – This herb has been in use from the middle ages as a stress reliever, as well as sleep inducer. In fact, a study managed to prove that people who took around 600 mg of its standardized extracts were found to be calmer and more alert when compared to people who took just a simple placebo. Of course, while it is considered to be generally safe, there have also been studies that show how excessive intake of it can make one more anxious. In this case, always follow the instructions and always begin your intake with a small dose. Lemon balm can be taken as a capsule, tea as well as tincture.

So there you have it, just a few examples of simple herbal remedies that should help you manage your anxiety and allow you to get better sleep at night.

Conclusion

Thank you again for purchasing this book on natural herbal remedies and how they can greatly enhance your life!

I am extremely excited to pass this information along to you, and I am so happy that you now have read and can hopefully implement these strategies going forward.

I hope this book was able to help you understand the vast world of herbal remedies and how you can use them to your benefit. Also, if you know of anyone else that could benefit from the information presented here please alert them of this book.

The next step is to get started using this information and to hopefully live a happier, healthier and much more fulfilling life!

If you know of anyone else that could benefit from the information presented here please inform them of this book.

Finally, if you enjoyed this book and feel it has added value to your life in any way, please take the time to share your thoughts and post a review on Amazon. It'd be greatly appreciated!

Thank you and good luck!

Preview Of:

<u>Honey And Natural Remedies</u>

Incredible Ways For Using Honey, Apple Cider Vinegar, Lemon, And Many More Natural Remedies To Boost Energy And Restore Health!

Introduction

I want to thank you and congratulate you for purchasing the book, *"Honey And Natural Remedies - Incredible Ways For Using Honey, Apple Cider Vinegar, Lemon, And Many More Natural Remedies To Boost Energy And Restore Health!"*.

This book contains insight on the amazing and healthy uses of Honey!

In your search for treatments for some common health issues such as a simple abdominal ache or the common cold, you may have encountered expensive, yet ineffective solutions. I truly understand how it feels to spend a lot and end up with basically no benefits from the artificial remedies. This is where honey enters the picture.

In this book I have presented some of the basic uses of honey. Along with these uses are some of the most promising benefits that honey individually can offer you, as well as, uses of honey in concert with other ingredients. Should you decide to use the sweet liquid with some of the other interesting ingredients you can readily find in the kitchen, here is a short teaser of some of the dynamic combinations. In this book you will find honey paired with combining agents such as: nutmeg, cinnamon, apple cider, cane vinegar, and lemon extract.

Hopefully, the information that you can get out of this book can help you come up with natural, affordable, and safe alternatives for some of the most common pressing problems that you have to face, medically or otherwise.

Thanks again for purchasing this book, I hope you enjoy it!

Chapter 1: Pure Honey And Its Uses

Pure honey is one of the most beneficial food items that nature can give you. In fact, people from the past highly valued this food not just because it helped them satiate their hunger, but also because of its medicinal properties. Today honey is used and supplying many benefits that you cannot readily acquire from other raw food sources. This book will let you in on some of the uses that pure honey can bring once you consume or apply it. Because of the plethora of uses and benefits of honey I did not want to over-complicate this book causing the reader to search with a fine tooth comb for the answers he or she is looking for. So instead of writing it in a story like fashion I wrote it in a much easier format for the reader to find the use they are looking for. As an added benefit to the reader, this will also act as a much easier reference guide in the future. I hope you enjoy some of the amazing benefits and uses as much as I have!

Face Wash

Using the substance as a facial wash is one of the typical applications for pure honey that can bring a lot of benefits to your skin. You simply have to combine warm water with a small drop of honey. Then, you may directly apply the mixture on your face and gently massage it in using circular strokes. You should keep in mind that the strokes should be done upward and outward. After you have conditioned the skin, thoroughly wash the honey off your skin with cool water. Washing off the honey with cool water will also result in helping your face keep its moisture.

Hair Shine

Honey was even used during the ancient times in history to enhance hair luster. To do this, you need to mix a teaspoon of honey to one quart of water, preferably the water should be warm so you can dilute the sweet substance easily. You may directly apply the mixture on your hair and let it soak indefinitely. In case you are wondering, you do not have to rinse off the concoction as you have already diluted it in the first place. Interestingly, the mixture can also help you calm the frizzles down found at the end of your hair strands.

Antimicrobial Substance

Honey can also be useful in cleaning up some fresh wounds and cuts. This sweet substance works in similar fashion as antibiotic creams. Because pure honey is antimicrobial by nature you may directly apply it on your minor burns, cuts, and some scrapes. You may do this using a clean hand or an applicator. After applying the honey you may want cover the wound using sterile gauze or bandages.

Anti-anxiety Agent
Mixing pure honey with some of your favorite tea brews can enhance the calming effect of these warm drinks. Honey can further improve the effects of the drinks as far as anxiety relief is concerned. You may also add this substance to other drinks such as lemon juice and ginger ale. In fact, you may even combine these two latter liquids with tea and honey to make another interesting drink. The ratio of each component will purely depend upon your own preferences.

Bath Essential

If you happen to be a fan of bath oils and salts you may want to consider using honey as an organic substitute. To do this you need to combine three tablespoons of pure honey to bath water. If you want to really go wild you can add in the combining agent - olive oil (around two tablespoons) and you have an interesting twist to your bathing experience! If you use this mixture regularly you will enjoy a conditioned and well-moisturized skin, not to mention a pleasant odor as well.

Precaution

These are just some of the benefits from using honey. If you are unsure about your body's reactions once you apply honey on your skin or ingest the fluid internally you should seek consultation with your physician first. Most likely the doctor will advise you to undergo a series of tests for an allergy to honey, these tests will take around two weeks to complete. For this procedure, you may be temporarily restricted from consuming honey and other types of similar substances. In case the physician discovers that you have some allergic reactions to the sweet substance, you should refrain from consuming honey all together until your doctor says otherwise. If you still want to do so, you may ask your physician to make the necessary adjustments to help you out. The take home here is that if you have any doubt at all whether or not you are allergic or may have an allergic reaction to honey or any other ingredients in this book, it is best to find out for sure by seeking the proper medical advice by a professional.

Thanks for Previewing My Exciting Book Entitled:

"Honey And Natural Remedies: Incredible Ways For Using Honey, Apple Cider Vinegar, Lemon, And Many More Natural Remedies To Boost Energy And Restore Health!"

To purchase this book, simply go to the Amazon Kindle store and simply search:

"HONEY AND NATURAL REMEDIES"

Then just scroll down until you see my book. You will know it is mine because you will see my name "Sarah Brooks" underneath the title.

Alternatively, you can visit my author page on Amazon to see this book and other work I have done. Thanks so much, and please don't forget your free bonuses.

DON'T LEAVE YET! - CHECK OUT YOUR FREE

BONUSES BELOW!

Free Bonus Offer: Get Free Access To The www.LuxyLifeNaturals.com VIP Newsletter!

Once you enter your email address you will immediately get free access to this awesome newsletter!

But wait, right now if you join now for free you will also get free access the "Secrets of Becoming A Meditation Expert – In 7 Days!" free Ebook!

To claim both your FREE VIP NEWSLETTER MEMBERSHIP and your FREE BONUS Ebook on the SECRETS OF BECOMING A MEDITATION EXPERT IN 7 DAYS!

Just Go To:

www.LuxyLifeNaturals.com